My Journey
through Breast Cancer

by
Jan Brearley

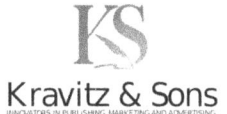

Kravitz and Sons LLC
1301 Farmville Blvd, Suite 104
Greenville, NC 27834

© 2025 Jan Brearley. All rights reserved.

No part of this book may be reproduced, stored in a retrieval system, or transmitted by any means without the written permission of the author.

Published by Kravitz and Sons LLC.

ISBN: 979-8-89639-324-5 (sc)
ISBN: 979-8-89639-323-8 (e)

Library of Congress Control Number: 2025912047

Because of the dynamic nature of the Internet, any web addresses or links contained in this book may have changed since publication and may no longer be valid. The views expressed in this work are solely those of the author and do not necessarily reflect the views of the publisher, and the publisher hereby disclaims any responsibility for them.

Table of Contents

The Silent Predator 1
Dear Mother 2
I Just Want You to Hold Me 3
CANCER 4
Chemotherapy Prayer .5
Angels Unaware 6
Gentle Giants 7
Losing Hair 8
Forgiveness 9
My Knight in Shining Armor 11
I Found a Bra Today .13
The Last Christmas 14
To My Blood Donors .17
One Day at a Time 19
State of Affairs 20
Happiness 22
Graduation Day 23
Embracing Cancer 24

The Silent Predator
By Jan Brearley

You came into my body today.
You came in with just one small cell.
Quietly, painlessly, you went unnoticed
As you gathered your troops and converted my cells.
Life, as it was, continued as usual
While your army was growing in my body.
"Seek and destroy"
Was your motto.
Then, when your "army" got large enough
You were discovered.
I discovered you with my very hand.
I felt you, I touched you, I feared you.
Cancer sought me out.
Looking to destroy me as it had my beautiful Mother,
Taken long before her time.
God, she fought the fight of faith
But in the end the cancer army won out,
Leaving me an orphan.
I declare to you today, Cancer army,
You will not win!!
I will take back my life!!
I will prevail!!
I may no longer have my breasts,
But I have the life inside me that you cannot claim!!
Never, no never!!

Dear Mother

By Jan Brearley

I feel your strength, dear Mother.
From your heavenly seat on high.
You, who walked this very path so long ago,
You, who fought and struggled and suffered,
Only to lose in the end.
I so missed your presence at my college graduation,
Following in your footsteps as a nurse.
I missed you on my wedding day,
The births of you precious grandsons,
Your great grandsons,
These past thirty-seven Mother's Days.
I feel your presence with me now,
When I need it most,
Strengthening me,
Encouraging me,
Sharing my burden,
Giving me hope for the future.
We can do this dear Mother,
We can beat this cancer together,
Hand in hand, Linked together forever.
Your strength is mine, United as one.

I Just Want You to Hold Me

By Jan Brearley

Why are you avoiding me?
Why don't you want to help me through this?
Why must I beg for you to be there for me?
I just want you to hold me.
You said you loved me
For better or worse
Do you remember?
I just want you to hold me.
I know I'm not sexy without breasts.
I know my hormones are raging
My emotions tattered.
I just want you to hold me.
This is my life
Why can't you understand?
I am fighting for my life!
Please help me
I just want you to hold me
When that first drop of chemo enters my veins
I just want you to hold me
While my hair is falling out
I just want you to hold me
When I'm feeling good and happy
I just want you to hold me
Forever in your arms
I need you
I just want you to hold me
Please.

CANCER

By Jan Brearley

You thought you took my breasts
But I gladly gave them up to save my life.
You thought you took my hair
But I gladly allowed it to fall out to save my life.
You thought you took my strength
But the weaker I felt on the outside just made my inner
Strength rise up stronger.
I may cry
But I am strong.
I may feel sorry for myself
I am allowed.
You thought that you had ruined my life,
But I have used you.
I have used you to renew old friendships,
Make new ones.
To heighten my empathy for the faces I see weekly,
To fully feel the warm sun on my face,
To truly hear the rustling wind through the trees,
To savor the taste of freshly baked banana bread,
To feel the softness of my kitten's fur,
And the gentle nudge of my horse's muzzle.
How lucky I am.
To have been given the opportunity
To stop the madness of this thing we call
"Life",
And experience the simple joy
Of just living.

Chemotherapy Prayer

By Jan Brearley

Lord, as I receive my chemotherapy today,
I envision this medicine cleansing my body of any
leftover cancer cells,
Washing me from head to toe in
Your peace and everlasting righteousness,
Resetting my metabolism back to where it was when
I was twenty-five years Old,
Breathing precious life back into my mind, body and spirit,
Allowing me to live a better life now and forever.
I thank you for this now, Father, in Jesus' name, Amen.

Angels Unaware

By Jan Brearley

Thank you, God,
For giving me an angel unaware today,
Embodied in a big black nurse named Key.
Her radiantly smiling face,
And tender hug around my neck,
Made me feel that I mattered.
"We're gonna get you through this, honey",
She stated, as if she knew this for a fact.
I realized
That she had taken the hands of so many before me,
With great success.
Key had risked
Getting attached to the throngs of people
Who passed through her door
Knowing that there may not always be a happy ending.
Yet she continues to extend herself
With hope, assurance, and confidence
Accepting nothing less.
I pray a special blessing today
For my angel unaware.
May her beacon of light
Continue to shine on us
In the very midst of the darkness
As we swiftly recover
From this cancer.

Gentle Giants

By Jan Brearley

They seemed different today,
Not sniffing my hair, as usual
But instead, sniffing my chest
Where my breasts had been removed.
From the cancer.
Gentle giants
Tenderly, gently sniffing my chest
As if they knew that I was infirmed.
Tears flooded me, but it was okay.
My gentle giants remained steadfast
Allowing me to cry the tears of loss.
I knew that they would stay here with me
As long as I needed their support.
Such gentle giants
These horses of mine.

Losing Hair

By Jan Brearley

It happened today.
Fifteen days after my first chemotherapy
The shower drain was full
Of my beautiful auburn, brunette hair.
I gently scooped it up
And placed it in the trash.
There was more
While I was styling my hair.
I knew this was coming.
I don't know which was worse
Surrendering my breast
Or my hair
To the greater good.
I refuse to admit
That cancer took my breasts and hair
Surrendering them gives me more control.
After all
It is for the greater good
Of the whole.
That I may live for many more years
Watching my grandchildren grow up
And enjoying the simple pleasures
That until now I had missed.
I thank God for the treatment I am receiving
To save my life
And make it better
For me, and everyone around me.

Forgiveness

By Jan Brearley

Forgiveness is a choice
Not a feeling.
I once heard it said
"Unforgiveness is like you drinking poison
And expecting someone else to die".
Forgiveness is not easy.
Letting someone else off the hook,
When they don't deserve it.
When they have wronged you, hurt you.
Forgiveness is for me.
It allows me to live more fully.
Out from under the veil
Of holding someone responsible
For their actions, words.
After all
Isn't that God's job?
"Forgive our trespasses
As we forgive those
Who trespasses against us".
He knew.
He knew how burdened down
We would become
If we didn't forgive.
There is a difference, however
In forgiving
And allowing someone to walk all over you.
Loving yourself
Knowing yourself
Putting yourself
first Is not a selfish act
But a courageous one.
Sometimes forgiving yourself

Is the hardest of all.
But if I choose to forgive myself
I, too will be let off the hook,
That does feel good.
As I go through this day
Help me to forgive myself
Along with others
For the injustices
That I am faced with
So that my life may radiate
Peace, joy, and tranquility
Now and forever.

My Knight in Shining Armor

By Jan Brearley

I wanted him to be my knight in shining armor
I wanted him to ride in on his white horse
Sweep me off my feet
And carry me to safety
Where I would not be touched
By this cancer.
But he couldn't.
No one could.
So, instead
I punished him.
I punished him
Because my Dad left me
When I was a baby.
Over and over
I punished him.
After all
I couldn't do it very well
Punish my Dad.
He was long in the grave.
But my husband was ever by my side.
What the hell made him stay?
Maybe, I unconsciously tried
To make him leave me
As my Dad had.
But, he didn't leave me.
He stayed by my side
For the past thirty-three years.
Maybe he really does love me.
I want to stop punishing him
Today.

I want to forgive my Dad for leaving me
Today.
Oh, God
I was looking everywhere
For my knight in shining armor
And here he was
Right in my own backyard.

I Found a Bra Today

By Jan Brearley

I found a bra today
From my life before
I thought I had done away with then all
Before my mastectomies
But there it was
Stuffed way back in my sock drawer.
Maybe I unconsciously stowed it away
To remind me of what I was
Before the cancer.
I should have tossed this one too
But I couldn't
I held it ever so gently
Turning it over and over in my hands
Remembering my beautiful breasts
I could still smell their essence
Even though I know it had been laundered.
I cried for my loss today
The part of my body I will never have again.
I will probably cry again.
When I drag that bra out.
Somehow, that's okay.
I need it
To help me remember
My life before.

The Last Christmas
By Jan Brearley

It's Christmastime again.
I hear the Christmas music
Playing on the radio
While I am driving
To my chemotherapy appointment.
As I pass the mall
Cars are spilling
From the parking lot
Of shoppers
Buying treasures for loved ones.
It's Christmastime again.
Once again I remember back
To the last Christmas
That I spent
With my precious Mother,
While she lay dying
In a hospital bed
From the dreaded disease
That is now mine.
I was twelve years old
That last Christmas.
We opened our presents
With our mother
My brother and I.
While she lay dying
In her hospital bed.
I could see a little more
Life slipping from her
Each new day
I tried to be happy
As we opened the presents
That she had chosen for us

Long before
She came to lay in this hospital bed.
The nurses buzzing
In and out,
Routinely gathering my Mother's vital signs.
I will be strong for her.
But inside I am terrified.
Terrified of living
Without my precious Mother.
Without her guidance and care.
"I'll Be There" by the. Jackson Five
Was recently released as a forty five record
And I carry it with me
Wherever I go
Using it as a mantra.
"Whenever you need me,
I'll be there." Believing that she will be there.
Now it is my turn
To battle this dreaded disease
Just as my Mother had.
I so want to be happy this Christmas
But the memories flood me
As always
During this time of year,
Memories of the last Christmas I spent
With my precious Mother
In the hospital
As the cancer gradually claimed her body
Leaving me alone and vulnerable.
I will use my strength
And yours, Mother
To sustain me
Through this difficult time.
And if I'm here next Christmas
I'll let go of the sorrow
Of the last Christmas with you.

And begin new memories.
Memories of gratitude
For each new Christmas
That I can spend with my beloved family.

To My Blood Donors
By Jan Brearley

To
Blood Donor #WO35208202806
And
Blood Donor #WO35208202809
I would like to thank you both
For your selfless contribution
To enhance the quality of my life.
Being a nurse,
I was terrified at first
Upon learning that I needed a blood transfusion.
Terrified of what undiscovered disease
Lurked in the cells
Of a stranger's blood.
I watched carefully
As your blood filled the IV tubing
Getting closer and closer
To my body.
My nurse prayed for me,
Asking God to give me peace
And He did.
I, in turn, prayed for you.
I prayed
That God would richly bless you.
Bless you in your coming and going,
Your waking and sleeping.
I feel the strength of your blood, now
Coursing through my veins,
Giving me determination
To fight this cancer.

Determination that had dwindled
From the weakness caused
When the chemotherapy
Killed my precious red blood cells.
I know I will never know your names
Dear blood donors
But I will never forget you.
You will always be a part of me
Together Amen.

One Day at a Time

By Jan Brearley

Living one day at a time means:
Living today.
Being consciously present every moment of today,
Without worrying about tomorrow,
Or wondering how it will turn out.
Living one day at a time means:
Trusting that God has my life planned,
Therefore I don't have to think about it.
I just have to rest,
In His peace, Knowing that there will be a path before me,
When it is time for me to take the next step.
Knowing that He has made provisions for me along the way.
A place to rest,
Food to eat,
Protection when I need it.
God has provided all of this for me.
It is mine But only by living one day at a time.

State of Affairs

By Jan Brearley

I listened to six songs
While on hold with my insurance company,
Only to discover
That I had not called the correct number.
"I will gladly transfer you",
which she did
To another automated woman
Who couldn't understand me
When I gave her my social security number,
Even after I entered it
With the keypad!
Aren't we suppose to avoid stress
When we have cancer?
Isn't that the first thing
They tell you?
Healing cancer is mind, body, and spirit.
Okay, I'll try it again
This time with a glass of wine
In my hand.
I'm feeling a little less stressed
When my insurance company tells me
That the doctor's office
Has "coded" the bill wrong
And that's why I now have a nasty letter
In my hand
Threatening to turn me over
To a collection agency.
I have cancer!
You're threatening me
With a collection agency?

It would be comical
If it weren't such a pitiful state
Of what our world has come to.

Happiness

By Jan Brearley

No one can make you happy.
That is something that you must do for yourself.
Why has that taken me a lifetime to learn?
Why am I trying to make everyone else happy
When that is something they must do?
And yet, it leaves me feeling
Resentful, frustrated, angry.
In order for me to be happy
I must put myself first.
I must put my happiness first.
But that seems selfish.
Something I learned growing up.
Putting yourself first,
Is not lady like or Kind and gentle.
You must put everyone else's
Needs, wants, and desires
Above your own,
Until you are a raging idiot,
Because everyone has what they want
Except you!
I finally get it.
Not all of the things we learned in our youth
Are true.
God, help me
To unlearn the other "truths"
In my life
That have not served me
And have actually kept me in bondage.
Amen.

Graduation Day

By Jan Brearley

It's graduation day!
Not from high school
Not from college
But from chemotherapy!
They place my graduation hat on my head
They play the graduation march.
I am finished!
Time to get on with my life.
What exactly does that mean?
What can I retain from this experience
That will make me a better person?
How can I continue to appreciate life?
Cherish the little things
As I go back to work
And reenter the world
That I have temporarily been absent from?
Help me, God
To daily appreciate
My life
My health
My family, friends
The beauty of Your earth
With every awakening day.
Amen.

Embracing Cancer

By Jan Brearley

Cancer.
At first I feared you,
Then I hated you,
Now I have accepted you,
Even embraced you,
As a part of my life.
You plucked me from my existence
And placed me on a new path.
An unknown path,
Fraught with surgeries
Chemotherapy,
The fear of dying,
So much out of control.
And yet, I have found peace there.
I have made new friends,
Seen another side of the world,
One that is not always pretty,
But in its midst
There is peace
If one looks for it.
There is beauty, and joy.
Life goes on.

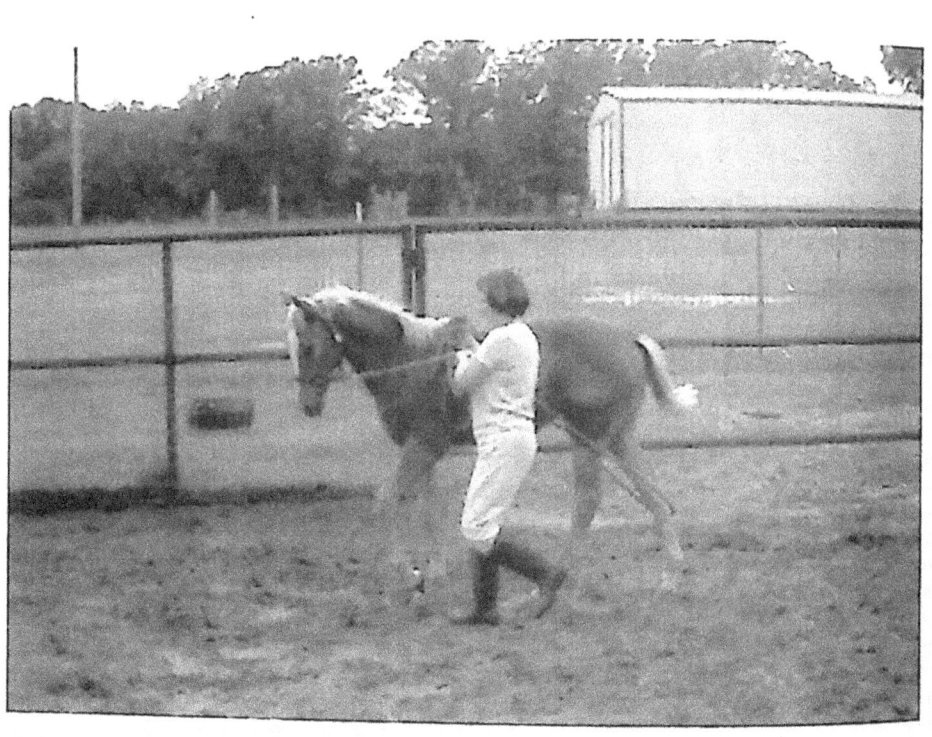

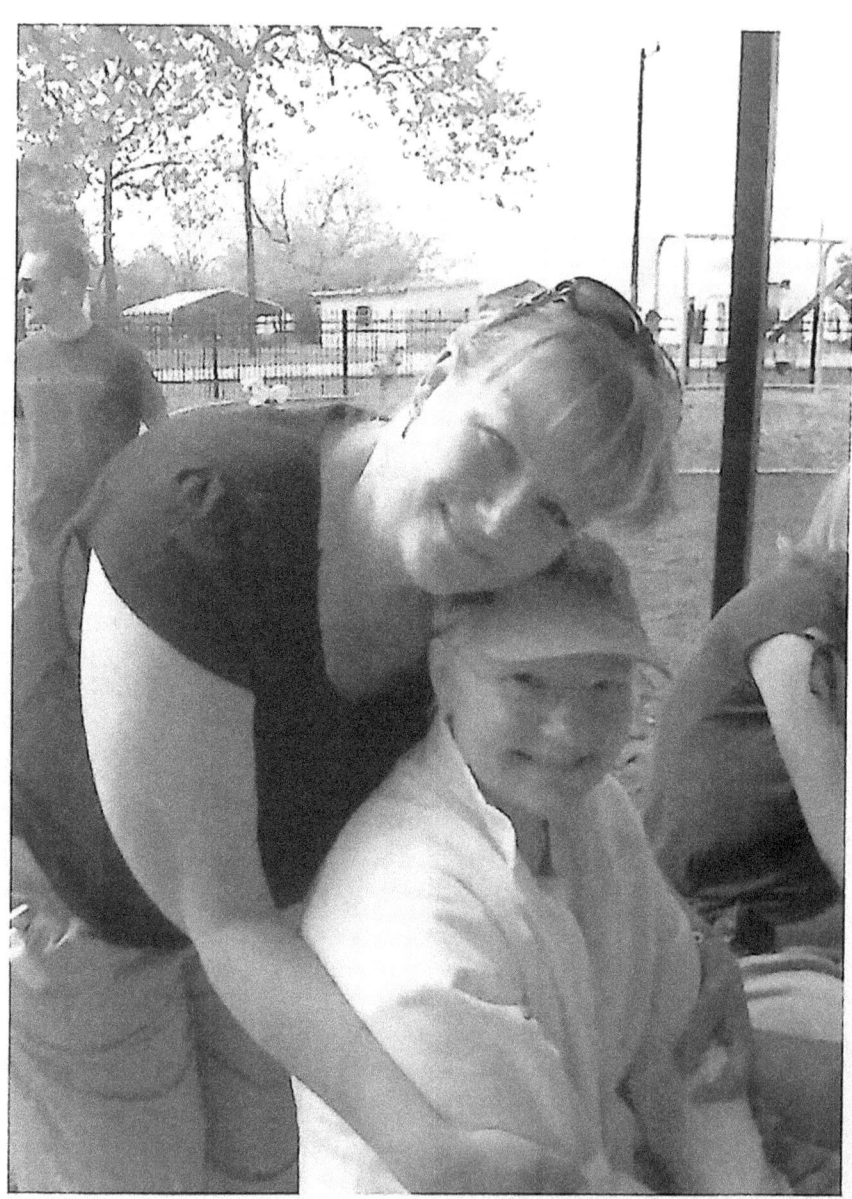

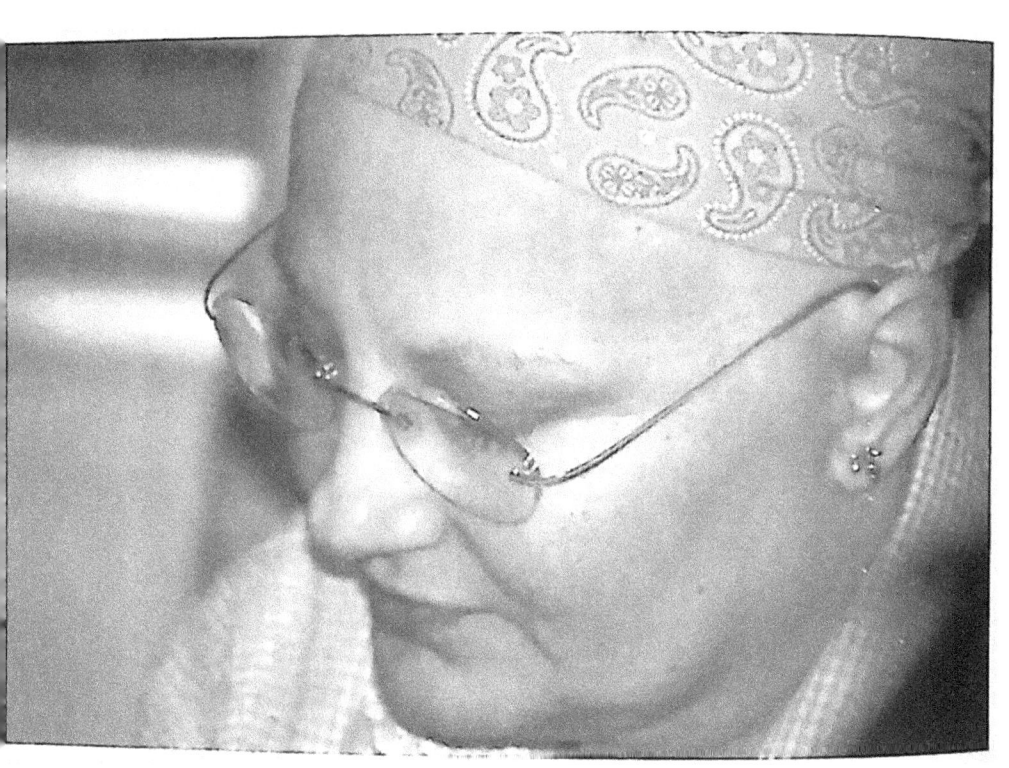

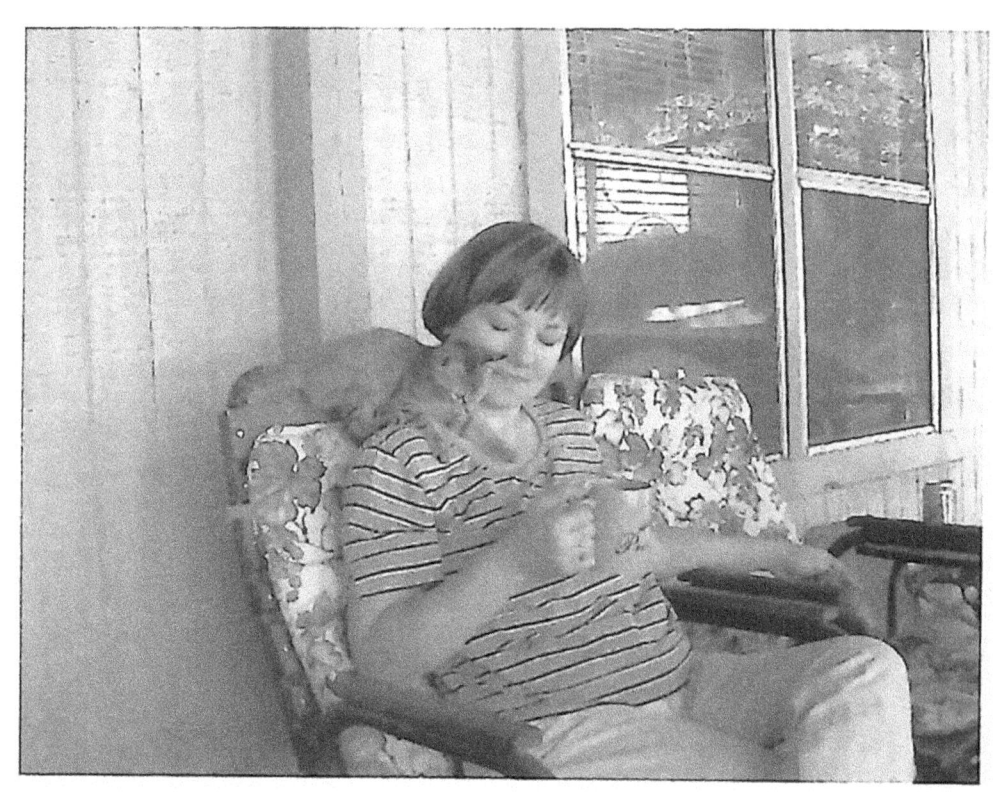

www.ingramcontent.com/pod-product-compliance
Lightning Source LLC
Chambersburg PA
CBHW030010040426
42337CB00012BA/727